THE BATTLES of TEN WOMEN
Short stories that put faces on cancer in women

I.C. OZED-WILLIAMS

Foreword by Dr. S.A. Adewuyi
(Consultant Oncologist, A.B.U.T.H,
Shika-Zaria)

THE BATTLES OF TEN WOMEN

By I. C. Ozed-Williams. FOTTBanner 2022

AUTHOR: I. C. OZED-WILLIAMS

Published in the United States of America
ISBN 979-8-9872427-8-0 (sc)

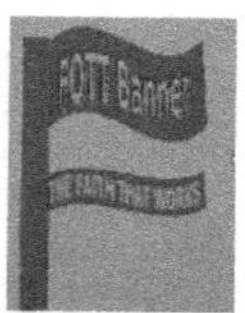

© 2007 by FOTT Banner Productions
P. O Box 213, Linthicum. MD 21090
e-mail: icozedwilliams@gmail.com

FROM THE AUTHOR…
These are stories about real people. If you recognize any of them, it is because it might be someone you know – a relative, a neighbour, a colleague, a friend, the friend of a friend, or maybe even a distant acquaintance. It might even be yourself! The things described here really happened and continue to happen. The names used here were not the actual names, except in one instance – Isobel Kuhn. Some of the stories are the story of more than one person but they were merged and highlighted to bring out a certain point.

In these our times, cancer is very real. A lot of attention is being paid to People Living with HIV/AIDS, to Tuberculosis, to Leprosy and so many other ailments. Even Malaria is getting a good share of the government's attention now, but the people living with, and dying of cancer do not seem to get enough attention. It is as if the disease is being over-shadowed by these other ones. The public remains pathetically unaware of it, and do not know what they can do to prevent the ones that are preventable, or where to go for help. Kudos! - to organizations like The Nigeria Cancer Society, The Society Against

Breast Cancer, Operation Stop Cervical Cancer and a few others. They are doing their best, but they are like just a drop of water on parched ground. They need more support before their efforts can become really meaningful.

The World health Organization has taught us that the prevention of a disease can be done at three levels:

1. *Primary Prevention: Not allowing the disease to occur at all, by avoiding certain habits, and espousing others.*
2. *Secondary Prevention: Prompt and adequate treatment of any disease at its early stages before complications develop.*
3. *Tertiary Prevention or Rehabilitation: getting back one's life after the problem has been dealt with, and learning to live positively with any residual effects from the disease itself, or from the treatment of it.*

The story of dealing with cancer can benefit maximally from this advice.

The stories in this book did not all end well. Some of them in fact ended very tragically. The major aims of this book are first to inform the public about some of the faces cancer would come with. The ones described here occurred in women. There are cancers that affect men only, some affect both men and women alike. Even children are not exempt. The public should know that cancer can be avoided, recognized early, and help obtained to battle it.

A second aim in writing this book is to give people a glimpse into the world of cancer patients, and their immediate care-givers – their relatives, their friends, their colleagues at work, and sometimes the doctors and the nurses that care for them in the hospital. May this terrible disease never happen to us or to someone that we know. However, as long as we continue in this world, unexpected things tend to happen. We do not have total control over our lives. We should learn to sympathize with those that are less fortunate. We should also receive sympathy if ever we are in those same shoes. An Igbo adage says that you mourn yourself the day you mourn another human being! We are all the same under our skins.

The final aim of this book is to bolster the spirits of those that have the disease right now or have ever had a hint of it. Hang in there! Do not succumb! You are not alone! There are people suffering right along with you and rooting for you. Any extra day that you gain is a victory by itself. We are certain that we shall all die someday but most of us do not know how, and nobody knows when. Look at cancer this way: at least you know how death is planning to come and get you. Well, it has made the mistake of giving you notice unlike other sudden deaths. Take time to plan these remaining days. Leave a lasting legacy. Arm yourself and do not be idle. Do not crawl into yourself and die before it has even come knocking. Use the time left to do what you have always wanted to do, and what you are able to do. Who knows, death may turn cowardly at the last minute, and postpone its harvest day. A cure might be found just as you are waiting. It has happened before.

We are rooting for you!

Your Fellow Pilgrim

FOREWORD

Cancer is as old as medicine itself! It is a genetic disease in its origins but not necessarily hereditary. Its hallmark is uncontrolled growth. There is no part of the body that is not susceptible to cancer (apart from nails, teeth and hair) although there is striking international variation in the occurrence of most cancer types. Despite its being genetic in origin, the epidemiology is influenced by both environmental and genetic composition of the individuals. This is responsible for the variation in the pattern of cancers seen in the different continents of the world. Cancer is real and no age group, sex, or social class is spared.

There is paucity of knowledge on factors implicated in the aetiology of cancers. This paucity of knowledge is not restricted to the general public alone. It is found even amongst the health workers. This may account for the widespread ignorance in the populace and poor response to the various screening programmes aimed at diagnosing cancer at very early stage or even preventing progression of pre-malignant condition to malignant lesions. In developing countries and especially in this environment, people view cancers from different perspectives. It has different names and means different things to different people. The understanding of many is that cancer is caused by evil spirits. As such, the treatment of choice is generally a spiritual approach. In the developed countries, on the other hand, there is now an unprecedented decline in rates of cancer-related death as a result of awareness and early diagnosis, prompt treatment, and availability of sophisticated medical equipment. The opposite is the norm in this environment. Ignorance, late presentation, apathy for orthodox treatment, and poverty are the prevailing factors.

The incidence of cancers in developed countries is dropping drastically for the past two decades due to successful screening programs. On the contrary, the incidence and prevalence is rising in most African countries. This reflects the attitude and practice towards screening and the persistence of socio-cultural factors that put the population at risk.

Cancer therapy is becoming increasingly complex. Today, most solid tumours, even very early cancers, are treated by more than one modality. This multidisciplinary and multimodality approach to treatment requires the input and coordination of multiple specialists. To complicate matters even further, often more than one therapeutic option exists. The rationale of multimodality approach is that success is cumulative. Thus, the combination of these treatment modalities produces better results than any option used alone. The resultant effect of multimodality and multidisciplinary treatments is a significant improvement in disease free survival, overall survival, and quality of life of the patients.

The choice of treatment modality for a particular disease depends on a lot of factors including the stage of the disease, patient's performance status, histologic result, natural history of the disease, available expertise, patient's acceptance, and financial status. These factors influenced the prognosis and goal of therapy. The various treatment modalities in the treatment of cancer include surgery, radiotherapy, chemotherapy, hormonal therapy, and immunotherapy. Others include Cryotherapy, hyperthermia, and photodynamic therapy. Historically, surgery was the sole method used for treating cancer. However, with the introduction of ionizing radiation and the development of anticancer medications, cancer therapy has rapidly progressed to involve the careful integration of an extensive array of therapeutic options in the treatment of primary, recurrent, and metastatic tumours. As a result, the cancer surgeon no longer works alone, but is part of a multidisciplinary team involved in the treatment of most solid tumours.

All hands must be on deck to prevent cancers. The general populace and health care providers must be health conscious, live a healthy lifestyle, seek help appropriately and to involved in health education of the people. They must also encourage screening programs.

DR. S. A. ADEWUYI
MBBS (ABU), MCPS, FCPS, FMCR, FICS. CONSULTANT & LECTURER   CLINICAL & RADIATION ONCOLOGIST

RADIOTHERAPY AND
ONCOLOGY CENTER *AHMADU
BELLO UNIVERSITY TEACHING
HOSPITAL, SHIKA – ZARIA,
KADUNA STATE, NIGERIA.*

DEDICATION:

To all women everywhere, anywhere:

Surely God had a special plan in making women special as they are!

Contents

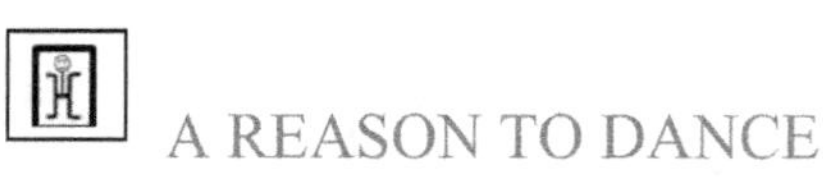 A REASON TO DANCE

– Jenny

The first time I saw Jenny, she was just too obvious. It was in church, and she was dancing too hard - harder than every other person around, and that was something. Even though it was a church of well-to-do folk where dancing was usually done in a gentle and dignified manner, it was a special occasion and people were dancing a bit too hard. However, Jenny outstripped them all. She was just so full of life, and dancing quite exuberantly.

The next time that I saw her, it was in a hospital. No, she was not the patient herself, she was the doctor! She wished to get the opinion of another doctor for her patient who was very seriously ill. The distraught wife just would not let Jenny go. Jenny was so compassionate. She was not just rendering the services of her skills and her training, but she was also ready to share her time, even her very soul! I was so intrigued that I just had to inquire about her.

It turned out that Jenny was forty-five years old. She had been married for twenty years, and had no children of her own – well, no biological children of her own. She had so many other children of different classifications. She had adoptive children, foster children, spiritual children, and so on.

About two years before I met her, Jenny had discovered a lump in her left breast. Being a doctor, she had immediately gone for a Fine Needle Aspiration Biopsy (FNAB). A needle was introduced into the lump, and something withdrawn in the syringe. The thing had been tested by histology. The result came out equivocal. It was neither here nor there. It could not be said for sure whether the lump was Benign (innocent), or Malignant (a cancer).

Jenny was advised to take antibiotics for a week, and then have the lump removed afterwards. About a month later, the lump was still the same size but had become quite painful. Her fellow doctors felt it was as a result of the FNAB. However if the truth were to be fully told, it was that they were being quite emotional in treating their colleague. None of them wanted it to be anything too bad. That is why doctors are told not to treat those that are close to them. They were also humans, after all, and their emotions would tend to becloud their judgements.

But thank God that Jenny had no such illusions – or perhaps she did, accounting for that one month interval. She insisted on having that lump out. It was not doing her any good by remaining a part of her body anyway. She was not afraid of surgery nor of anaesthesia. It was probably a lot of bravado. Put like that however, the doctors had to perform the surgery. The lump was removed and sent for histological tests. "It is a colleague's specimen", her doctors insisted. "We want the result out as soon as possible so that we can reassure her."

But the result when it came out was far from re-assuring. It was cancer!

Everybody panicked. The doctors panicked! Jenny's husband panicked! Jenny's parents panicked! The whole hospital panicked! Her church panicked! Even her neighbours panicked! Jenny herself was also panicked! It was as if Jenny was already dead. Fortunately the major players recovered their senses on time. Bravely, within the same week, Jenny went to have the second surgery. Her entire left breast was removed. The cancer did not seem to have spread. The breast was sent for further histology however. Everybody waited with bated breath. The result seemed to take forever to come out. When it finally did, there was a general sigh of relief. It was cause for celebration. The cancer indeed had not spread. Jenny still had to take a few medications as a precaution. That was all.

"This is over five years since all this happened" Jenny concluded. "Look at me now. I could have died but I am still alive. Not only am I alive, I can move, I can dance, I can sing and I can laugh. Tell me why shouldn't I be praising God? Those that dance in a gentle manner do so according to how God has blessed them but He has blessed me so obviously so I must dance very obviously! God has indeed given me so many reasons to dance so why shouldn't I dance to praise Him?"

Why indeed? This is now about seven years since she told us that story. She is still alive, still dancing, and as far as I know, the cancer has not recurred.

Myths and Mythologies

Cancer of the breast is the commonest cancer that affect women world-wide. It is also very deadly. Here are a few myths that surround the disease, and the real truths that explode the myths.

MYTH I – Cancer of the breast affects women only.
THE TRUTH –*Cancer of the breast can affect men too, and in men it tends to be more deadly than in women because without the cushioning effects of the fat of the breast that women have, the cancer tends to penetrate the chest wall or the skin faster.*

MYTH II –Only fat women ever get cancer of the breast.
THE TRUTH –*Skinny women tend to have cancer of the breast as well with equal frequency. The initial lump may feel bigger because of the fat, but slim women are not exempt. Obesity though carries a higher risk for breast cancer.*

MYTH III –People that breast-feed well never get cancer of the breast.

THE TRUTH *–Breast-feeding does not confer any special advantage to developing or not developing cancer. However, it would probably be easier to detect a lump in the breast that is often handled so that treatment can begin before it spreads.*

MYTH IV *–Cancer of the breast happens to only married women and those that have ever had sex.*
THE TRUTH *–Cancer of the breast can happen to anybody. It is just easier to detect in the breast that is HANDLED MORE OFTEN. This, incidentally, can prevent death from the disease.*

MYTH V *–Family Planning methods lead to cancer of the breast.*
THE TRUTH *–There are different family planning methods and many of them would not affect the breast. However, breast changes were noticed in mice that were given some of the family planning injections, in a dose that was fifty times the amount that human beings usually get. For this reason, any woman that ever had a breast lump removed is advised to choose other methods of family planning*

(other than the injections). Again, those that choose the injections, the pills or other hormonal methods of family planning are advised to go frequently for medical check-ups. It is not just enough to just continue these method without adequate medical supervision.

MYTH VI –Only old and menopausal women ever get cancer of the breast.
THE TRUTH –*Young women in their child-bearing years also get it. In them in fact, it rages like a wildfire or a storm especially if they get pregnant. (See the next section).*

MYTH VII –Cancer of the breast can be totally prevented.
THE TRUTH –*Until the cause is known for sure, cancer of the breast is not totally preventable. Happily, dying from it can be prevented especially if it is detected early, treated promptly, and adequately*

MYTH VIII –Hot water baths tend to relieve cancer of the breast.

THE TRUTH *– There are some treatment methods that are based on delivering a lot of heat to the cancer cells. The same amount of heat will also promptly kill normal tissues so it is not a treatment that can be applied to the whole body. It is not as simple as a hot bath, wet-towel compresses, nor even hot water bottles. However, it is said that soaking in a bathtub of hot water can relieve some of the pains of cancer. Theoretically though, it could also dilate the blood vessels, and encourage a quicker spread of the disease.*

MYTH IX *–**Cancer of the breast can be transmitted to a breast-feeding baby, or by close contact.***
THE TRUTH *–It has not yet been discovered that there is an infective agent in cancer of the breast, unlike in the cancer of the cervix. However cancer tends to sometimes run in genes. The sisters, daughters, nieces, aunts, and other female relatives, of a woman that have had cancer, are at an increased risk of developing cancer of that, or other types.*

MYTH X –Cancer of the breast means inevitable death.
***THE TRUTH** –This is not true at all. Just keep reading. In any case, everyone must die one day. It is definitely not everybody that has cancer of the breast that dies of it. Some die of some other things before the cancer can get them. Early treatment can achieve a full cure. Long remissions have also been known to occur. With modern treatments of cancer now, one can even hope to live for many more productive years!*

MYTH XI –Cancer of the breast always means mutilation of the body by removal of one or both breasts.
***THE TRUTH** –What about it? If removal of one or two breasts can save someone's life, is it not good? However, when the cancer is detected early, only the affected area alone can be removed and other modern treatment methods then applied. (See Appendix)*

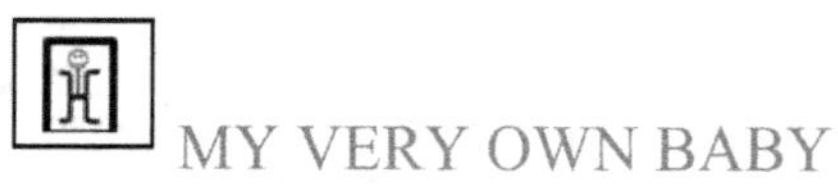 MY VERY OWN BABY

– Tutu

The naming ceremony was done in the hospital, and what an occasion it was! It was not the first time that determined parents decided to hold the occasion anyway because either the mother or the infant was unfit to go home yet. Even so, this one was with a difference! Whereas other parents made their celebrations low-key because of the environment, these parents were determined to make it as loud and as clear as possible. They had not gone to the extent of hiring a live band nor other noise makers, however. Nevertheless, they had hired many chairs and canopies. A lot of people came from outside the hospital, turned out in their beautiful and multi-coloured festive clothes and tall headgears. The hospital workers also came, those that were currently on duty, those that had gone off duty, and those that would be coming to resume later. The hospital security staff decided to turn a blind eye. They even joined in the festivities.

There was a lot to eat and to drink. Despite the festive mood, there was not a single dry eye in the gathering. However, these were tears of happiness. At long last, Tutu had a baby! The baby girl got eighteen names! They were eighteen well-thought-out names. The names were expressing praise and glory to God. They were names that had been in reserve for years because this day had been so long in coming.

Yes, Tutu now had a baby and it had taken her twelve years to finally have it. Tutu had a lot of things including a very sweet disposition. She came from a very affluent background. She had married into wealth, though for love's sake. She had a first-class degree in accounting, a master's degree in Business administration and worked with a very prominent bank as the assistant branch manager. She had very doting elder brothers, admiring neighbours, nieces and nephews. She had colleagues that hung on her every word. Yes, Tutu seemed to have it all, except for a baby!

She had gone through twelve years of hospital tests at home and abroad. She had even tried the modern reproductive methods for a test tube baby. Her husband, ever patient had gone along with her. He had not ever considered taking a second wife though this was culturally acceptable. He loved Tutu that much.

Tutu on her part portended to love her life so much, as well as the people in it. She was more often counting her blessings than mourning her woes. She always felt sad of course whenever any of her friends or her relatives invited her for yet another baby-naming or dedication. She never allowed these weigh her down for long. In fact, she felt more hurt when she was not invited. She was neither bitter nor jealous but was rather always so zestful.

When Tutu started feeling ill therefore, everybody was surprised. It was so untypical for her to be overcome by any illness. Her physician tested her for all manner of illness ranging from common cold to resistant malaria, and even typhoid fever. Although the test titres were only borderline, she still received treatment because she was still not feeling "Herself". At last out of desperation, he sent her for a specialist opinion. It was in trying to remember the date of her last menstruation that Tutu began to suspect that she might be pregnant!

The doctor examined her and sent her for several tests. Lo and behold, it was confirmed! Tutu had become pregnant despite not having been on any special treatment for over a year. In fact, she joked that she was on a permanent break while trying to gather herself. And then she was pregnant, unexpectedly pregnant. Tutu was jubilant! Her doctor was jubilant! Her husband was jubilant and so was every other person that knew Tutu!

"You must register for the antenatal clinic at once", her mother had insisted. It was at that first antenatal visit that a lump was discovered in Tutu's right breast. The doctor assured her that it might mean nothing! "But it's better to be sure before it becomes too late."

Tutu subjected herself to FNAB without thinking twice about it. However, the result came out –MALIGNANT!

What to do now? A conference was called, including the doctors and members of Tutu's family.

The situation was explained: Tutu really must have surgery to survive. The entire left breast had to go, and thereafter, there might be need for more extensive operations. She also had to start on cytotoxic medications. It was explained to them that the surgery posed some limited risk to the unborn baby, but that the medications would pose a definite risk to the baby!

Everybody was perturbed, except Tutu herself. She had read it all up and had already decided that she would subject herself to the surgery. She would have the breast out. The dangerous medications could be started after her delivery.

Tutu was scheduled to deliver by operation as soon as the baby was mature enough. She went into labour before the scheduled day and had her baby. That they were in the hospital on the day of the naming ceremony was not because of anything the baby had, it was that Tutu was being worked up for further treatment. The baby also had to be fully introduced to artificial feeding. Till she started on the dangerous medications, Tutu insisted on fully breast-feeding her baby.

At the naming ceremony, her husband ended his speech by saying, "God has rewarded our twelve years of patience. If He has seen us over that mountain, we know that He will be there for us as we climb over the mountain of cancer as well."

No wonder there was not a single dry eye at the ceremony!

⬚ <u>Babies and Cancers</u>

Some of the most heart-rending decisions that are ever made are when to choose between terminating a pregnancy because there is a cancer that needs to be treated, or allowing a pregnancy to continue, knowing that every precious moment the cancer may be spreading beyond where it can be treated, thereby shortening a woman's life!

Cancer of the breast especially has a most curious relationship with pregnancy. One of the medications used in treating cancer of the breast is also a fertility medication. Some patients on it get pregnant unadvisedly. Again, one of the hormones that support pregnancy also supports the growth of the cancer. Thirdly, one of the ways of containing cancer of the breast is to remove the ovaries (where the eggs come from in the first instance in order to make a baby). Failure to do this sometimes would cause the cancer to reach the ovaries, and from there, spread like wildfire.

If a pregnant patient is noticed for the first time to have cancer of the breast, the problem usually is what to do with the pregnancy. Outside of pregnancy, the patient is well-advised to use a very reliable method of contraception if the ovaries had not been removed by operation or knocked off by other means. The dilemma still arises when they become pregnant anyway. Mostly the moral question is not just as simple as not wanting to commit abortion. There is also the question of the mother's life. Should doctors deliberately shorten the woman's life?

If the cancer was found out by the time the baby was matured enough to survive outside the mother's womb, delivery is usually hurried up —by induction of labour or by Caesarean section. Treatment is then commenced for the mother immediately. For immature pregnancies, the case is totally different!

*There is no easy way out. Recently, there have been pointers to the fact that terminating the pregnancy did not necessarily prolong the mother's life. Sometimes, the treatment is commenced anyway, and the baby allowed to take its own chances. The truth is that **MOST** treatment methods are invariably harmful to the baby. The pregnancy will definitely* *abort, or the baby be born with defects. The baby also would have a greater chance of developing cancer later in life, especially of the blood.*

However, breast surgery on a pregnant woman is a safe treatment option for the baby at any time of pregnancy (See Appendix).

*Whatever has to be done in any case, the patient **MUST** be a part of the decision. In fact, the final decision rests with her, not with her doctor, not with her relatives, not even with her husband. As long as she is in her right mind, the final decision must rest with her! In fact, it is known that some women that would have died tended to live on sheer will alone till their babies were safely born. However, the plight of a motherless baby is also not so pleasant. Every woman should strive to survive for her children for as long as possible!*

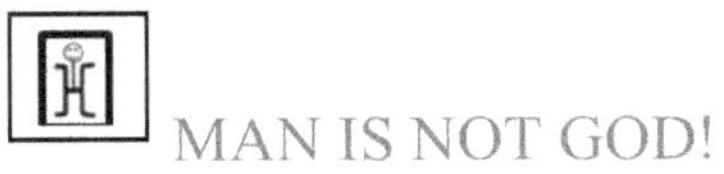 MAN IS NOT GOD!

– Ifeyinwa

"That," said the old consultant "is my oldest girlfriend!"

Well, he always referred to all his female patients as his girlfriends. The only exceptional qualifications this particular patient had was the attachment of the word "oldest". We all wondered and became interested. We waited in anticipation of a story, and we were not disappointed. He began:

"We did Ifeyinwa's case about twelve years ago. I had inherited her from my senior colleague. I remember the first day we saw her at the clinic. She had this lump in the breast that had caused the nodes in her armpits to swell. The pathetic thing was that the node in the other armpit was also swollen. This was a sure sign that the disease had really spread. My senior colleague told Ifeyinwa that she had cancer of the breast, and that it had become very advanced. As Ifeyinwa left the clinic, she was weeping piteously. We all felt very sorry for her, but there was no gentle way of telling her. The next week, she came for the clinic with her husband as if she needed his moral support. He seemed more upset than her. He kept asking for what could be done for his wife. How much longer was she expected to live?

In those days, the miracle treatments we know now were not available. Those that were available were not affordable. To obtain them were very difficult and cumbersome and required travelling. However, as the man kept pressing for answers, we had to refer them to the chief surgeon.

"We will take off the more affected breast," he told them. "Thereafter we shall do the most that we can to keep her comfortable. This thing has really eaten deep. It has probably invaded her lungs by now. On the average, we expect her to survive for about six months, give or take a few weeks."

Ifeyinwa was devastated. She kept asking over and over "What will I do with my four children? Who will I leave these children to?" She was not asking of these anyone in particular. She was not really expecting any answer.

Her oldest child was just sixteen years, and the youngest only six. Ifeyinwa herself turned forty just that year. The doctors and nurses were all filled with compassion. We practically neglected all the other patients to console Ifeyinwa.

Her husband started scolding her angrily. He kept telling her, "Woman, control yourself! Stop disgracing yourself! Stop all this noisemaking!"

They were harsh words, but we understood that people in shock said and did all manner of paradoxical things. We forgave him and comforted him too. It was not till the day of Ifeyinwa's surgery that we saw what the man really meant. The usual party of anxiously waiting relatives was made up of Ifeyinwa's mother and her elder sister. Her husband was not there! We asked about it.

Ifeyinwa started to say something, and then stopped. "Oh!" said her mother, "He will be coming later".

"Why are you not telling them the truth?" Ifeyinwa's sister cut in angrily. "He is not likely to come later at all. He travelled to the village today for his traditional wedding to his new wife."

We were stunned! How callous can a person get? It was true he had been told that his wife of eighteen years had only about six months more to live. How could he not have waited till she died before replacing her? What was the hurry in getting the new wife that he had to attend to the festivities on the day this other wife was to undergo surgery?

Ifeyinwa's surgery went uneventfully. While she was in the hospital still recovering, the husband came with the new wife to visit her once. The major burden of caring for her apparently rested with her mother. For the fact that she came daily to visit her with the children, we also understood that the children were staying with her while their father was on honeymoon or something of the nature.

A month after her discharge when she came for her routine follow-up, we were all looking morose. It was Ifeyinwa's turn to console us. Our chief surgeon, the one that had told her and her husband that she might have just about six months to

live, had died of a ruptured appendix just the week
before.

About six months after that initial diagnosis,
Ifeyinwa came to the clinic as usual. She was
looking quite chipper! "You must all come to my
thanksgiving party to celebrate with me," she said.

"What has happened?" we wanted to know.

"Two things she answered happily, "One is
that I am still alive even after the deadline I was
given. The second is that last week, my husband and
his new wife died in a car accident while coming
back from the village."

Macabre reasons to celebrate? Maybe! But
we totally sympathized with her and we all attended
the lavish celebrations.

"All of that was about twelve years ago," the
old consultant concluded. "Ifeyinwa is still alive and
is even a grandmother so many times over now. She
still attends our clinics once a year, as close as
possible to the date when she was supposed to have

died. The cancer has not resurfaced yet and we are
very hopeful."

🎓 <u>**Is That Possible?**</u>

Did Ifeyinwa really have advanced cancer of the breast or was it a mistaken diagnosis?

This is a very pertinent question. However, knowing the calibre of the doctor that told the story, and how thoroughly such things are usually investigated before pronouncements are made, she probably did have advanced cancer. But even if she did not, and it was a case of misdiagnosis, does that not make the story even more interesting?

But cancer behaves in a most interesting way. When patients are being treated, doctors give what they call a five-year survival rate, as if five years is a lifetime! But come to think of it, a lot of things can happen within one year, so that five years is really of great significance. Within this time, the patient may die of some other cause, but if the disease can be held at bay for five years, it is almost as good as cured.

Many times, especially with treatment, many cancers just tend to stop growing. Sometimes they tend to have become dormant – gone to sleep. These are called "REMISSIONS". Nobody knows for sure what can cause the cancer to suddenly re-awaken but when they do, they tend to then grow with renewed energy. Sometimes, another remission can occur, most other times, not. A remission can last for weeks, for months and sometimes even for years. It is as if the individual and the disease have called a truce and agreed to co-exist.

Maybe what Ifeyinwa had was just a remission but imagine what changes would have taken place in that intervening period: all her children at least had become independent. She had even become a grandmother. All her problems as she lay dying, waiting for the six months she had been told had all been over-taken by events.

That is why doctors appear very reluctant to answer ALL the questions that patients put to them. Man is not God, and no one can say for sure what will be after now. The most doctors can tell their patients is: "Academically speaking... from what has happened to other patients... we think that... However,..."

Pity the doctors!

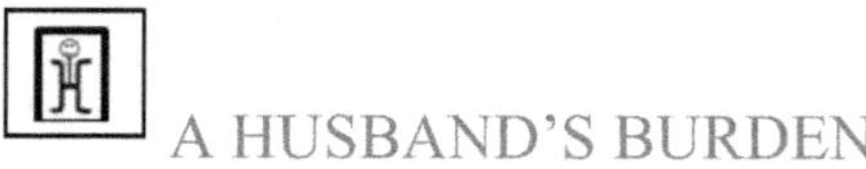 A HUSBAND'S BURDEN

– Magajiya

She was very aptly named – Magajiya – a leader, a queen! She was a born leader, one of those that came naturally endowed, not just to be a leader among men, but also among women as well. She was tall and stately, and as intelligent as she was beautiful. The emotions she awakened among people – old and young alike, male, and female alike, was not that of envy nor competitiveness, but rather of awe, of reverence, of servitude even! Although her mother, her sisters, and her brother were shadowy figures in the background, no one was really acquainted with her private life. Her private life did not unduly intrude into her very prominent public life.

Magajiya's husband was also a leader among men. Indeed, it was not known for sure whether Magajiya was her given name, or a name she had acquired as a result of her husband's various public positions. With the typical shadow that enshrouded such prominent figures, it had been rumoured that she was the one that had shot her husband to prominence with the wealth endowed from a previous marriage. Other rumours had it that this was not so. He was the one who had been married several times previously to different rich women whom he had divorced just to be with Magajiya only.

But rumours were rumours – just a series of unsubstantiated stories that were circulated among eager ears. What everybody knew for sure was that both of them were in a liaison that pleased them very much. Their marriage was definitely not the first for each of them. Even their detractors acknowledged that they definitely complemented each other and were very happy in the relationship.

And then a problem developed! It had all started innocently enough. Magajiya noticed that she was having a very profuse vaginal discharge. At first, she disregarded it. She felt that every woman had these things from time to time. And then the discharge increased, causing her underpants to be sticky and uncomfortable. And then the colour changed from a creamy white to yellow. Next, the odour became very terrible! She felt that whenever she entered a room that everybody would definitely perceive it despite her costly perfumes.

She was quite embarrassed and finally decided to talk to her official doctor about it. The doctor ordered swab tests and placed her on a course of antibiotics. The odour reduced, the colour lightened, but the volume of the discharge if anything, increased!

As if there was not already enough problems, she noticed that she tended to bleed on days she was not expecting to, even when she had just completed her monthly menstruation. This disturbed her normal activities a lot. Worse still, she tended to bleed very profusely after sex. This was the last straw! Sex had always played a very important part in their marriage. It always formed a meeting point in their very busy, separate schedules.

Discussing the discharge, she was having with another person was one matter, but discussing the intimacies she shared with her husband with a third party was definitely most embarrassing – almost a taboo! Finally, however, Magajiya picked up enough courage to tell her mother about it. The poor old woman became instantly alarmed. She had a friend who had such complaints and had eventually slowly died of cancer. She insisted that Magajiya see a doctor immediately. Magajiya chose to fly out of the country and use a doctor that was relatively a stranger. Her worst fears were confirmed: she did indeed have cancer of the cervix!

With their worst fears confirmed, it seemed that everybody discovered a hidden source of strength – Magajiya herself, her husband, her mother, in short everybody that was in the know. There were modern medications, operation, and radiotherapy. All manner of advances had been made in the treatment of this cancer. However, Magajiya's illness had quite advanced before any treatment could be started. She was rapidly going downhill.

The discharge increased with a vengeance. It was so offensive that no one could stay for long in the same room with her. No amount of antibiotics had any effect whatsoever. The room was constantly being sprayed with air fresheners, but this sometimes tended to add to the oppressive atmosphere.

The bleeding became almost constant. She had to be transfused on several occasions. She took to wearing infant napkins instead of the customary pads just in an effort to curtail it. No reasonable treatment could be commenced because her blood levels were always too low. Finally, however, a modified form had to be given her just to contain the bleeding. This seemed to help but very soon afterwards, she lost control over holding back her urine and faeces. She leaked urine and faeces constantly.

Magajiya probably finally gave up the day it became obvious that her husband could not stand being in the same room with her for long. In her usual pragmatic way, she understood them all. She was more or less very much a burden. She could not move about by herself, not just because of the weakness caused by the constant loss of blood but also because the cancer had also invaded her backbone. She knew that she was dying. It was just a matter of time. When she was told that she needed further transfusions to keep going, she firmly refused. She asked to be transferred to the hospital. The hospital refused her admission on the basis that there was not really anything they could do for her as an in-patient that they could not do for her while she was at home. Magajiya even understood that. She would have liked to die at home, surrounded by her family if not by her friends but she knew she was too much of a burden there.

At last, she asked to be taken to a hospice. The cost of care there would be expensive, but she felt this was one last luxury she could afford, one last favour she could do her loved ones.

And so, at last Magajiya, the Queen, the leader among men and women, great daughter, and beloved wife, died – the husk of her former self, a smelly mass in a cold hospice room but surrounded by the cards and flowers those that had loved her and remembered her good days had sent. Her husband had just the one comfort: "I was with her as she breathed her last!"

⬛ <u>The Wrath of God?</u>

Cancer of the cervix (the "neck" of the womb) is one of those cancers that the world is struggling to eradicate. It is a sexually transmitted disease. It is virtually unknown among the celibate, but very common among the following:

- *People that have more than one sexual partner*
- *People whose sexual partners have more than one sexual partner*
- *People who started having sexual intercourse at a very tender age*
- *People who have other sexually transmitted diseases.*

Smoking by itself does not cause cancer of the cervix, but it enhances the onset and the spread of the disease. This is true, not only of the active smokers, but also of the passive ones, that is those that are constantly in the company of those that smoke and are forced to continually inhale the stuff.

It has now been established that certain types of the Human Papilloma Virus, a close relative of the HIV, is what is responsible for causing cancer of the cervix. Efforts are now being made to develop vaccines against it which should be given to both males and females. Men do not have cervices, and therefore would not develop cancer of the cervix. However, it is known that any man who had ever lost a wife to cancer of the cervix, is likely to lose another one the same way too.

One of the most terrible things about the cancer of the cervix is the smell! Other cancers also smell as they are destroyed, the living tissues around them die, and as infections develop around them. However, because of the location of the cervix, the difficulty in reaching it while bathing, the bacteria and other micro-organisms that live naturally in that area, and other factors, they tend to smell very terribly.

There are now active, affordable, widely available means of screening for cervical cancer. Every woman that is sexually active or has ever been, and especially those that have, or whose partners have or had more than one sexual partner is advised to utilize it frequently. In most countries, it is done yearly from eighteen years, or three-yearly for those who have consistently had negative results but have remained with just one partner, who himself also has had no other partner. The frequency increases or decreases depending on different circumstances.

This is one cancer that can be fully cured if detected early enough. Unfortunately, the utilization of the screening facilities is very low indeed, even among health workers. By the time symptoms develop, the cancer is already established. Even then, it can still be cured. The major problem is that people are rather shy of discussing their symptoms.

Recently, the HPV vaccine has been introduced for prepubescent children. At first, it was available for girls only. Now it is advised that even boys should get it as well. For one, they will be the consort for those girls. It is not unknown for wives of the same man to die of cervical cancer. It is sexually transmitted after all. Again, it was found to also prevent penile cancer.

Let us work together to drive out this one cancer from the lives of   women – and of men!

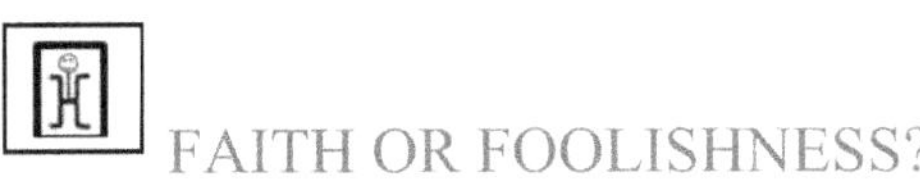

FAITH OR FOOLISHNESS?

– Shola

Shola had gone to the hospital for something totally different, but her doctor had offered her a free "PAP smear" as a part of an on-going program. Shola accepted. Going back the following week to check the result, she had been confronted with the verdict: ***"Developing"*** Cancer of the cervix!

"It's not my portion!" Shola declared. She went home and discussed it with her friends, her sisters, her neighbours, and any other person that cared to listen. She always concluded the story with: "They say that it is cancer of the cervix but that is not my portion! God cannot ordain cancer for me!"

They all listened to her sympathetically, and then also "reject it" with her. "Cancer is not your portion!" they said.

That is, all of them, except for Tolu. Tolu had been very good friends with Shola since they were little girls. They had gone to all their schools together, done most things together, and after marriage had found themselves living in the same city so their friendship had just continued. Tolu was very different from Shola in one very big aspect. Whereas Shola had always been the dreamer, Tolu was always very practical and very down-to-earth. It had caused them some disagreements in the past but the rift was never too deep to be healed. When Tolu had heard Shola out on this latest issue, she said, "What did they suggest you should do? Did they say it is treatable?"

"Oh! They offered me to remove my womb. Can you imagine that? They said that if I did that at this stage, it will not develop into a full-blown cancer."

"Oh! It is not even cancer yet. So why are you waiting until it develops into a cancer? Let them remove your womb if that will spare your life! What are you doing with the womb anyway? You already have six children as it is. You are not planning for more."

"Remove my womb? What are you saying Tolu? By the time I stand before God and He asks about my womb, what will I tell Him?"

Very practically Tolu replied, "That you had to sacrifice it in order to save your life. You think God does not know what you are passing through now? You think that He is even now not making a way of escape? Be reasonable. I think you are limiting God in your thinking."

"Exactly!" replied Shola. "I don't want to limit God in my thinking at all. He is going to prove Himself in my life. You will see that He is able to heal all things including cancer!"

"Oh yes!" Tolu pressed on, "But why do you want to dictate to Him the way that He should heal you? I think that it is enough of a miracle that they even discovered it now while it is yet very early and still treatable. Don't be foolish Shola. Go to the hospital immediately and fix the appointment for the surgery!"

But Shola was adamant. She would not be budged. Nobody in her family had ever had this kind of illness before, she argued. Bad things would not begin with her especially seeing as she is very special to God! She was so sure that the reason God was allowing this in her life was to demonstrate His favour upon her. He would use His healing of her for signs and wonders. After a rather loudly vocal disagreement, Tolu gave up on her and went home. She vowed not to set eyes on her friend again.

Shola went from one prayer house to another, one "Man of God" to another. She solicited prayers and sought miracles, wanting to move the hand of God, and to change the verdict. They made her do dubious things like drink water with bits of mysterious things dissolved in them. She had to fast for several days while sleeping in hygienically questionable places. She used incenses, holy water, anointing oil, and various coloured candles. And then she began to develop symptoms.

At first it was light vaginal discharge that steadily got heavier. The discharge became mixed with blood and was very bad smelling. The false prophets assured her that this was indeed her body trying to get rid of the disease. Special diets were prescribed for her. The highlight of these diets was that many things, especially proteins were prohibited.

The next time she saw Tolu a few months later, was quite dramatic. They bumped into each other at the market. While still going through the preliminary greetings of "Long time, no see", Shola suddenly collapsed in a dead faint! Tolu panicked. Acting on pure instinct she managed to get help to take her friend to the hospital, their uncompleted shopping forgotten. Fortunately, her hospital tracer card was found in her purse. Her records were dug up. While waiting for the doctors attending to her friend, Tolu called her own husband as well as Shola's husband. The latter arrived first but they were all together when the doctor, with a very grim face informed them, "I'm afraid she now has frank cancer, which is not being helped by her mal-nourished state. At this stage we cannot now operate. If we are able to build her up, she can still be cured by Radiotherapy."

"I will not undergo any such treatment," a much-recovered Shola announced from her bed. I

have heard how it finishes people's hairs –
eyebrows, scalp hair, and even pubic hair! I heard
that the diarrhoea and the vomiting it causes can be
unbearable."

Tolu looked at her helplessly, pleading with
her gaze but she said nothing. At least she agreed to
the blood transfusions. Knowing how stubborn her
friend could be, she took both their husbands outside
and tried very hard to appeal to Shola's husband.
"Please make her take the treatment," she begged.
"Think of what people will say if she died. They will
say that you stood aside callously and watched her
die. Please force her, do anything."

"What can I do? You know what she is like.
Make no mistake about it, I have talked and talked,
but she only gets very irritable whenever it is
mentioned. I have decided not to mention it
anymore."

Tolu continued to plead, with tears even. She
got so worked up that her husband intervened and
led her away.

To be fair to Shola's husband, he did try to see if there was a way he could commit her to receiving the treatment. The doctors pointed out to him however that his wife was a legal adult. She was in her right mind, and nobody could do any such things against her wishes. Tolu on her part also tried to get Shola's children to plead with their mother. It was all in vain. It was a big burden to place on children. Some obviously sided with their mum. The youngest had no idea what was going on. Shola's old mother and her sisters could convince her. Three months after she was discharged, Shola called Tolu one day to tell her that she was "Going Native".

"Going Native?" asked Tolu puzzled, "What does that mean?"

Apparently, someone had mentioned to Shola that a herbalist somewhere knew how to successfully cure the disease. At this stage, Tolu decided to shut off from Shola altogether. "To protect my sanity and deliver myself from further heartaches" she said.

And so, Shola began to go from one herbalist to another, one native doctor to another. She had not accepted hospital treatment because she said she believed absolutely in God's power to heal. Everything changed. A year later, she was leaking urine and leaking faeces. She was oozing very smelly stuff from virtually every pore of her body. Her flesh was rotting even while she still breathed. Her presence was an offence to everybody that was anybody at all, and those that were not. She lay at Death's door.

She sent for Tolu who had not seen her for a very long time. What Tolu saw hardly looked like a human being. Shola had shrunk totally. Only her abdomen was very grotesquely swollen. She looked nothing at all like the vivacious lady that had been her life-long friend. Her eyes were very dim and sunk into her skull. Her teeth stood out very prominently. Her voice was weak and rasping. Tolu leaned forward to hear what she was trying to say, trying very hard to keep from vomiting. She was unable to swallow her own spittle. She realised there was great anger in Shola's voice.

"I am dying Tolu," she said. "I am dying a very disappointed person. I have lost faith in men as well as in God. They have all failed me very woefully. I feel much cheated."

Tolu could not answer. She had so much saliva in her mouth. In any case, how do you begin to tell such a person she was the one who was failing God and man? Tolu left. About a week later, Shola died. Everybody, including her children, was so relieved. "It is best for her to go and rest", they said. What they really meant was that they too would rest from the burden of caring for her.

Two months later, her husband remarried. "I need help with the children," he explained.

The Horse and the Water

"You can drive a horse to the water," goes the common adage, "but you cannot force it to drink!"

Unlike the previous case where the cancer was not detected until it was too late, this person's disease was not only discovered early, but discovered when it was not even cancer yet. Various remedies were even offered at the different stages when it was still possible to cure it but she refused them all!

The society we live in would rather go for a big-time show than accept the ordinary and the mundane. This, even when the ordinary is known to be more effective. It is not always a problem of ignorance and illiteracy either. Even the so-called enlightened ones are part of it.

Doctors lament over patients that could have been saved but chose to try all alternative means and spend most of their resources. These alternative means are not cheaper either. Some are known to be very notoriously expensive. The patients then come back, for those that do. By then, it is too late for the doctor to be able to do anything.

Some patients go from doctor to doctor, trying to get a "Second opinion". A second opinion in the right context should actually mean that the patient goes to the second doctor, armed with a letter that explains what the first doctor had found and done so far. The letter should also say what he or she thinks the problem is, what could be done.

What these patients actually do is to hide all the findings of the first doctor to see if the new doctor would give a different opinion. They go shopping for the doctor that would tell them what their hearts would like to hear. These things they would like to hear is often not the truth. Of course, any reasonable doctor confronted with a fresh patient without facts and findings would have to begin afresh in order to come to some decisions. The result of all these of course is that precious time continues to be lost when action ought to have been commenced.

For those that eventually come back to their senses and listen to reason, it often comes too late. "Fortunately" for these people, medical ethics does not allow doctors to refuse to treat even such patients.

This story illustrates one woman's folly but it happens all the time. As we have opportunity, let us be among those that give positive counsel. "It is best to make hay while the sun is shining".

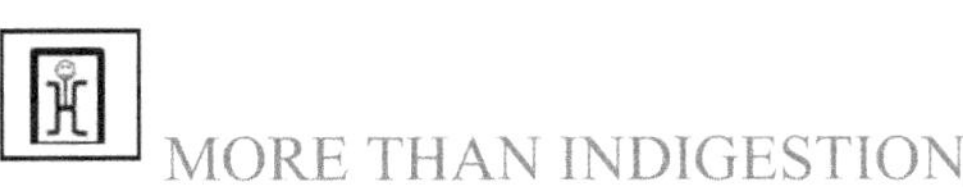 MORE THAN INDIGESTION

– Ojoma

If anyone should ask Ojoma, she would have said that all her problems started on the day of her Retirement party. She had so looked forward to retiring that when the day finally came, she felt she just had to have a party – and why shouldn't she?

She was the first of six siblings. She had suffered very much to raise all the rest after their mother died. Of course, her father had been a great help. With the power of hindsight, so had been her stepmother. However, her siblings had turned solely to her as their mother-figure. She had even married when she did, which was immediately after her secondary school, in order to provide a stable home base for her younger siblings.

In getting married at that time, she had hoped that it would enhance, rather than hinder her chances of pursuing higher education but one thing had led to another. She had had a profusion of pregnancies. There were childbirths and miscarriages. At the end she had eight more children to care for! Her husband was not a very rich man, so Ojoma had supplemented the family income by doing a lowly secretarial job in a private set-up at first. Later she landed her job in a government ministry. She still found the time to squeeze in sandwich courses and holiday school programs. No one quite knew how she did it all, but she did! At the time of her retirement, she had eight straight, well-educated, children. She had put in thirty-five years of civil service, and looked forward to the pension of a senior government officer. She did it all by the dint of hard work and steady progress.

And what did she plan to do after she retires from active service? "Ah! I will wake up by eleven o'clock every morning. I will have a long bath, and then go visiting. When one town becomes too boring, I will pack up my bags and travel to another town. I will get to become acquainted and re-acquainted with my children, grandchildren, nieces, and nephews. I will never allow anything to become routine in my life again!"

Such a grand ambition! Everyone she told would laugh! Yes, Ojoma deserved a lot of rest and leisure. However, by her very nature, or the dint of long years and habit, everybody was sure she was not going to sustain that kind of schedule for any length of time. "Sooner or later, we shall hear how busy and industrious she has again become."

But Ojoma did get one thing right very unwittingly: her life was never going to be routine again. Never!

After the retirement party, she complained of indigestion. "Nothing much," she said, "just an unsettling of the stomach. Maybe I sampled too much of something or maybe ate something that didn't agree with another, and they are having a fight in my tummy."

A friendly pharmacist prescribed antacids and anti-flatulence for her. She actually felt better after the medications. She proceeded to start enjoying the first weeks of her retirement. But then she began to feel increasingly restless. It was either her abdomen was too full of gas or food, but her abdomen seemed to be consistently full. Sometimes, it would be as if she was going to menstruate, but her menses had ceased over five years before. People suggested that perhaps she was suffering from the effects of slowing down in life. Ojoma took to taking long strolls and volunteering for almost any activity going on around her. These, at least helped to keep her mind off the problem but in actual fact, she began to feel constantly tired.

At first, over-the-counter treatments from the chemist near her house was giving her momentary relief. However, the time came when her husband decided that this was not enough anymore. Ojoma had never been one to complain or malinger. Even in her thirty-five years of civil service, she hardly took time off for the sake of ill-health. He decided that it was time they saw a doctor.

The doctor began again with all the treatments she had been getting from the chemist. She received mild medications to treat annoying problems like indigestion, constipation, aches and pains. He treated her for malaria, in case it was atypical malaria. In addition, he ordered for a barrage of tests all of which came out either normal or on the borderline of the abnormal. It was when she did not pass stool for three days and was doubled up with pain that he ordered an abdominal ultrasound scan. That was when they discovered that Ojoma had cysts in both her ovaries. Both ovaries were very much enlarged, especially for one who was no longer menstruating.

He immediately referred her to a bigger hospital. Ojoma had the benefit of being attended by doctors of different specialties. They carried out more tests, did an operation, and then asked for a family gathering. That was where they told them: Ojoma had cancer of the ovaries. It was also at the very late stages!

To be fair, nobody blamed any other person. Everybody blamed himself or herself for not finding out on time, especially her daughter who was a nurse. The doctors assured them that by the time she was having the first symptoms of indigestion, it was already too late anyway.

They were introduced to some very expensive and very

uncomfortable medications. They said these would help Ojoma live longer. Sacrifices were made. People ran around. Ojoma was a very compliant patient. She did all that she was asked to do but she got steadily worse. Six months later, barely into the second year of her retirement, she was dead. She was just fifty-seven years of age. She died as she had lived, with a joke on her lips: "I probably would not have been able to cope with all that free time anyway. I better try for a total change of environment."

A Silent Killer

Cancer of the ovaries is one of those diseases that will not give any signs at all until the disease has become "quite mature" and untreatable. There are some medications that are used to delay inevitable death after surgery has been performed.

Unlike cancer of the breast and cancer of the cervix that have screening methods, there is no easy way of screening for cancer of the ovary. Frequent ultrasound scan of the ovaries have been suggested. In truth, there is no typical appearances to watch out for. By the time any changes are seen, it may already be too late anyway.

Part of the problem is the location of the ovaries. They lie freely in the cavity of the abdomen. They have almost no contact with all the other important organs of the abdomen. At the same time, they are all bathed by the same peritoneal fluid. Another thing is that they have a lot of room to grow. That means that they may not show any undue signs or provoke any undue discomfort until they have become quite large.

Some people go to the length of removing their ovaries by operation once they feel they have the number of children that they desire. There is some sense in this especially if they have any first degree relative (sister, mother, or daughter) that had ever had any cancer at all, but especially cancer of the ovaries. Some do it if they have a particular implicating gene – BRCA. People that have this gene are more likely to develop cancer of the breast or ovaries sometime in their lifetime.

The disadvantage however is that the work of the ovaries is not just in making babies. They also produce some useful hormones, even after menopause. The work of these hormones includes the protection of the heart, the bones, the connective tissues, and other things.

After removing the ovaries, some of these hormones can be replaced as frequent medications but it is never exactly the same. Besides, every medication has its own side effect. At the end of the day, it all becomes a balancing act, and having to face and deal with any crisis as it arises. (See The Changing Tides by this   same author).

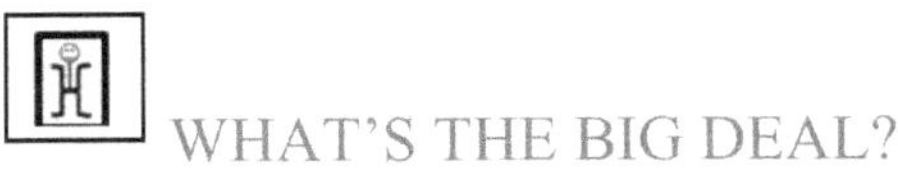 WHAT'S THE BIG DEAL?

– Rifkatu

Rifkatu was a cleaner in the hospital. She was the roly-poly, happy-go-lucky type that is well-loved by everybody. The other hospital workers loved her. So did the patients, and their relatives. Her cheerful nature attracted a lot of gifts from everybody. This was good for Rifkatu because she had nine children to feed. Her husband was just a lowly peasant who also did part-time labourer work for people at the government quarters. They barely survived but they managed to get along.

And then Rifkatu got pregnant again! She joked that it was so she could enjoy the mandatory three months maternity leave, and also get gifts from her friends and well-wishers. The people that knew her well knew that she was not very overjoyed about it at all. All the family resources were already over-stretched as it were.

However, the pregnancy was not progressing well at all. Unlike in her previous pregnancies,

Rifkatu was constantly sick. She vomited so much that she had to be admitted for some time although she would rather have stayed home. As she was entering the fourth month the problem ought to have subsided or stopped altogether. Instead, she took a turn for the worse. Her legs began swelling as that of someone that was already in her eighth or ninth month. Her face became puffy. When her blood pressure was checked, it was very high. This was totally unlike her other pregnancies. Rifkatu was re-admitted.

As if to relieve every one of the anxieties, the very next day, Rifkatu started bleeding and miscarried the pregnancy. She did not care to take a look at what had come out. She noticed though, that the doctors were unduly over-interested in the thing. They kept calling the more senior doctors to come and see till most had come to take a look. Rifkatu was more interested in being discharged. She was already feeling better. It seemed pointless to continue to remain in the hospital. The truth was that she was eager to return to work. Her family income was suffering without the augmentation of the gifts she occasionally brought   back from the hospital.

They let her go rather reluctantly. They explained that she had to report to the clinic weekly for blood and urine tests. She went twice. The doctors appeared unhappy about the results and were hinting at further admissions. Rifkatu fled. She did not show up for the next two appointments.

About a week after the miscarriage, she started bleeding. At first she thought it was the resumption of her monthly menstruation, but it lasted for only a day and stopped. She put it out of her mind. Over the next few weeks, she was bleeding on and off. This was not following any regular pattern. At last, she went back to the clinic to complain. They made her wait while they again carried out blood and urine tests. She was asked to also do a chest x-ray. When she was called in to hear the results of the tests, the first ominous sign was that she was facing not one doctor, but a team of doctors! They shook their heads gravely. It was a cancer, she was told. It was a cancer that could be cured, but a cancer, nevertheless. This cancer could also kill her. It was something that was related to the placenta.

This made no sense whatsoever to Rifkatu. Did the placenta not come out when she miscarried? When they all came to gaze and prod the thing that had come out, did they not see the placenta? In any case, if anything remained, it was their own incompetence!

Nevertheless, she allowed herself to undergo the rather painful experience of evacuation of the uterus. She agreed to be admitted for a week at a time every three weeks in order to receive some unpleasant medications. These medications caused her mouth and throat to be sore. They caused her hair to fall out. Besides all these, there was always, the constant prodding and bloodletting for tests and so on. It was all too much.

After the third admission, Rifkatu decided she had had enough! She deliberately did not go for the next appointment. She found out that she definitely felt better and stronger. She decided thereafter that she was not going to comply with the foolishness anymore. She had her work to do, and a family to look after. The doctors came looking for her. They even accepted her flimsy excuse that she had forgotten her appointment. She promised to come later. After that, she became more expert at dodging them. She got her other colleagues to collude with her. The doctors themselves also soon gave up the chase. They concentrated their attention on their more compliant patients.

And then one day, Rifkatu was admitted into the psychiatry ward. She was behaving abnormally and talking irrationally. Her husband and her oldest daughter who had brought her kept wringing their hands. They were unable to exactly and coherently tell what had happened to the bulwark of their home.

Later that night, the duty nurse noticed that Rifkatu was coughing up blood. The next day, her fellow cleaners came to visit her. About two days later, one of the Gynaecologists overheard one of them remark on how bad Rifkatu's condition had become. She was even unconscious. The doctor's ears pricked up. He asked a barrage of questions. Gathering the other gynaecologists, they went to pay Rifkatu an unsolicited visit at the Psychiatry ward. They reviewed her, and then invited the Psychiatrist to share with them. Rifkatu had a problem that had started from the womb but had now probably reached the brain. It was the placental-type cancer. Rifkatu had choriocarcinoma!

Some tests were done immediately, and their diagnosis was confirmed. They all put heads together and agreed on several things. One was that Rifkatu should be moved to the cancer ward, and appropriate treatments commenced. She could have chemotherapy or radiotherapy. First though, her blood and chemical profile had to be built up so she could tolerate treatment. That night, Rifkatu died without having regained consciousness. It was a very unnecessary death!

Master Deceiver

Dying from choriocarcinoma these days must be one of the most terrible disasters. This is one cancer that is very, very amenable to treatment. Not only can it be perfectly cured but the whole body system becomes restored to normal afterwards so that one can go on having babies if one chose to.

It is said that any woman that has ever been pregnant, no matter how long the pregnancy lasted, has a chance of developing choriocarcinoma. A case was even reported of a woman that developed it twenty years after her last pregnancy. Most choriocarcinomas follow an abnormal pregnancy called molar pregnancy. However, it could also result after a full-term, normal delivery, an abortion, a miscarriage, or even an ectopic pregnancy.

When choriocarcinoma presents "nicely", the signs and the symptoms would be clear. There would be irregular vaginal bleeding following a pregnancy that had ended "somehow". When it chooses to present "nastily", it masks itself and can mimic anything from Tuberculosis, to stroke (paralysis of one side of the body), to mental illness amidst so many other ways.

The good thing about choriocarcinoma though is that with adequate treatment it immediately disappears most times. A total cure is possible. Most times, operations are not even needed. Only injections or/and tablets are necessary! Most times only one type of injection is enough. In "resistant" cases, a combination of medications would then be required.

These medications have unpleasant side effects. However, once the treatment is stopped, everything would rapidly go back to normal. Most women are advised not to get pregnant for a while after stopping the treatment. This is so the side effects of the medications would not be carried over to their babies, and to monitor for any relapse in the disease.

Some women either cannot or would not heed these instructions. They still get pregnant in a shorter period. So far, no abnormalities have been reported in the babies but some of these babies were not followed up to   adulthood.

The use of radiation therapy has also been shown to be very effective against choriocarcinoma. This method of treatment has been described as killing an ant with a sledgehammer. Sometimes this is necessary but the effect on fertility might be worse than with simple medications.

Let us thank God for big and for small mercies. May we not despise His grace!

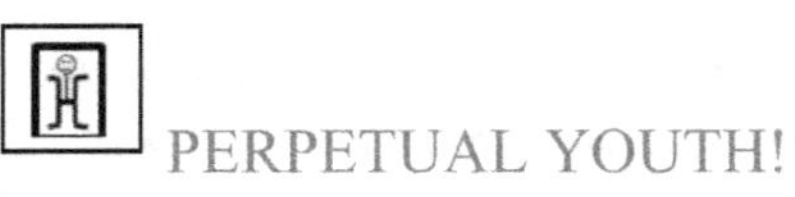

PERPETUAL YOUTH!

– Ejiro

Meeting Ejiro for the first time, no one would ever believe that she was sixty-five years old! In fact, meeting her with her daughters, who were in their mid-twenties, one immediately assumed that they were all sisters, daughters of the same mother. Ejiro would laugh at such mistakes mischievously. When asked the secret of her perpetual youth, she would always answer, "I just know how to maintain myself."

Ejiro really knew how to maintain herself. It was also not just by diet and exercise only like she was always trying to make people believe. Oh she dieted all right, and always went wildly into every food fad that came to her notice. There was a time she existed on only meat, fish and milk. Recently, she had become a virtual vegetarian. She would eat only fruits and vegetables!

As for exercise, she eagerly worked out at the gym daily. She was so passionate about fresh air that her room could become as chilly as a deep freezer on harmattan mornings, and Ejiro still would not allow the windows to be shut!

But apart from diet and exercise, Ejiro also had a passion for medication fads. She took medications to keep her slim. There were medications to strengthen her bones. There were medications to keep her teeth and gums healthy. She had medications to help her cope with menopause. This was in addition to all manner of food supplements, and so on, and so forth. One of her daughters once exclaimed, "Mummy, do you know that you take twenty-six capsules or tablets every day?"

To this Ejiro had cheerfully replied, "Oh, they are about thirty-two now. Some are for evening time, and I have run out of one or two. I hope to get new supplies in two days."

That was typically Ejiro! Her cosmetics were also something else. Seventeen years earlier when she was going through the problems of menopause, a friendly doctor had prescribed oestrogen supplements for her in

London. The next time she had requested for more, the pharmacy had refused to dispense it without a doctor's prescription. Desperately trying to reach the doctor, she had run into an old acquaintance who had told her that the medications were more easily obtainable, and with less stress at mainland Europe. "What's more," the acquaintance had said, "you can even get them as skin patches, in creams, or in lotions."

Ejiro had immediately gone to mainland Europe and found everything to be just as she was told. Since then, all of her cosmetics had to have the oestrogen supplements mixed into them! What Ejiro spent on maintaining herself was up to a small fortune, but she could afford it.

When almost twenty years after reaching menopause Ejiro started bleeding again, everyone just assumed it was part of her perpetual youthfulness. Ejiro herself however was quite perturbed. It was one thing to feel and look young, but the thought of the inconvenience of pads or tampons did not amuse her at all. Since she had to attend a social occasion that day, she nevertheless put one and carried on with her activities without paying it much attention. By the next day, the bleeding had petered out and stopped. Ejiro was grateful and just considered it an aberration.

A month later, the same thing happened. This time however, her daughter, who was a medical student, was around. She asked why her mom was sending for tampons. Ejiro explained. Her daughter immediately became alarmed. She spoke a lot of medical jargon, the essence of which was that bleeding from the vagina after one had passed menopause was very dangerous. Ejiro needed to get a medical check-up at once. They had to make sure that it was not cancer! She made arrangements for her mother to be seen at the hospital where she was being trained. The doctors all agreed with her verdict. A few tests would have to be done, but Ejiro should know that the best thing would be to remove her womb, cancer, or no cancer!

An immediate pelvic ultrasound scan showed that she had some moderately-sized fibroids. The fibroids could not possibly be the sole cause of the bleeding. They suggested a "D and C", in order to get specimen for histological tests. That was where Ejiro put her foot down, especially when they said this would be done while she was fully awake. She said that she would just hold on. She was due to travel to London on business in about a week, she told them. She hoped the doctors would not mind her getting a second opinion while she was there.

Privately, she remarked that she had no confidence in the indigenous doctors. "They are always knife-happy," she said. "They are forever wanting to cut and operate. Did I not have six children without anybody ever mentioning a fibroid? They are probably saying all that to hide their ignorance and incompetence!"

A week later she went to London. A hysteroscopy was done for her at a very handsome cost. There were also a few other tests that did not come any cheaper. Soon enough, she was called to hear the verdict. She had fibroids that were growing when they ought to have shrunk with menopause. The lining of the womb was also growing luxuriantly like grass in rainy season. All these pointed to the fact that she might soon develop cancer of the womb, or may already have an early stage of it. The most honest advice they could give her? *REMOVE THAT WOMB NOW, OR AS SOON AS POSSIBLE!*

Panicked, Ejiro agreed for her womb to be removed. She was too ashamed to go back home to have it done. Although she could ill-afford it at that time, she spent over ten times what she would have spent. At last, the womb was removed. Further tests showed there was no cancer seedling anywhere.

Today, Ejiro is free of cancer. Her daughter advised her to stop using all those cosmetics and medications, and to eat like every other normal person. She now looks much older than she used to look but she is at least much healthier, and she knows it. The other day somebody asked her if she still takes many medications. "Oh, I only two types of vitamins and two types of energy medications. I also take calcium and minerals supplements."

Some people never change their habits!

A Price to pay

There is a price for every benefit that we get in this world. It is reasonable that we should know the price before deciding whether the benefit is really worth it. Again, like every other thing, medical science keeps evolving. What had been declared as beneficial today gets declared as harmful in a few decades' time or less, and vice versa. A good example is "The Cholesterol" question. A few years ago, cholesterol was black listed as one of the leading causes of heart disease and every effort was being made to reduce the level of cholesterol especially with advancing age.

Today, it has been found that those whose cholesterol levels were not high enough in old age (especially those that had strenuously reduced it in order to prevent heart disease) are prone to degenerative brain illnesses like Alzheimer's disease. Recent research has shown that cholesterol is not a "Bad Guy" after all.

Everybody must be very careful of the food fads that they pursue. It is true that the secret of perpetual youth and longevity have not yet been discovered but life spans are longer now that they were before, like a century ago, or even a quarter of a century ago. This is despite mass accidents and disasters; air pollution and advanced methods of warfare!

The lesson still remains though. All things must be done in moderation, knowing that one must have to sacrifice one thing in order to gain another. It is still not possible to eat one's cake and still have it!

In any case who wants to continue to live in this flesh, on this side of eternity for too long? Even if it does not become too boring, one soon finds that the younger generation is coming up fast and claiming their own rights to the earth. They generally disregard the tested, older values. They introduce newer, stranger (and sometimes more workable values, if the truth must be told). They make the place more comfortable for themselves, and more uncomfortable for the older generation. However, after them comes another generation that would do the very same thing to them! But do not suppose that this much younger generation would be your allies. Rather than be on your side, they will regard you as archaic, museum pieces. You cluster their world and occupying unnecessary space. If you attempt to keep up with them, they will see you as an object of ridicule. They would rather have you as venerated memories! The world is like that. Think back!

One has to move on at some time. Choose very carefully and be kind to yourself.

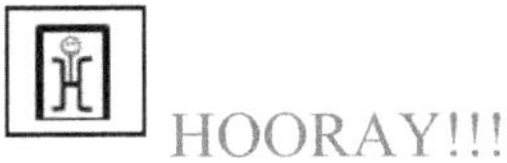

HOORAY!!!

– Eno

"Hey, Affiong, phone call for you!"

Affiong was only mildly irritated. It had been a fairly good day. The patients and their relatives had been fewer than usual, and considerably well-behaved. The nurses even had time for a tea-break in their common room. They were then in the midst of a lively political debate when the phone call came.

Affiong got up and went to the inner office to take the call. "Hello?" she said into the phone.

"Sister! Sister, it's me. It's Eno."

Eno was Affiong's younger sister, in fact, her only sister. Affiong was the first, then came four boys. After everyone had given up hope of their mother ever having another baby, Eno had come along. She was everybody's delight, especially Affiong's. The fifteen years age difference, and the fact that they often had to team up together against so many brothers brought them even closer. After wedding, Affiong had taken her sister to live with her. Eno had been like the eldest of her own children. She had gone home to her parents just a few years before to help nurse their mother through her final illness. She had stayed with their father to help him cope with the ensuing grief. As if she had not had enough tragedies, her fiancé proceeded to die in a car crash barely a week to the wedding.

Eno withdrew into herself. Gone was the sparkling mischievous girl. She hardly called anyone. She answered calls in short lifeless sentences. She never left home again, except to go to her job in a minor government ministry. At thirty-five years of age, nobody could force her to do what she did not want to do. Affiong was therefore very surprised to hear her actually initiate a conversation.

"How are you Eno? Is there a problem?"

"Well, yes. Kuffre said I should call you to let you know when I will be coming."

"Really?" asked Affiong. This was another surprise! Kuffre was the most thoughtful of all their brothers. If he suggested that Eno made the over one-thousand-kilometre journey, there was a very good reason indeed. "It's all right with us. Are you on leave?"

"Yes. They allowed me to take a leave. They said I could resume whenever I felt up to it" Eno answered tonelessly.

The alarm bells went louder in Affiong's brain. "What is it Eno? What is the problem?"

"It is too much to be discussed over the phone, Sister. I want to join the night bus today. I'll be there tomorrow morning."

"Okay. Call me when you reach the station. I will come to pick you up."

Affiong then spent the next eighteen hours tormenting herself with thoughts of what could possibly be wrong. Eno arrived early the following morning. When Affiong went to pick her up at the bus station, she got the first shock. Eno had always been fair, but now she was practically white with an unhealthy pallor! She could hardly walk. She moved as if the slightest breeze would blow her over. Even carrying her handbag seemed to require a lot of effort. Another passenger had to help her with her travelling bag, light though it was when Affiong took it over. When she got nearer, Affiong saw that she was panting as if she had just run a long race. Affiong embraced her and then just burst into tears.

As they drove back to the house, the story gradually emerged. She had menstrual periods that were so heavy and would not totally stop. Her underclothes were constantly stained with blood, some days more heavily than others. Terrible odours followed her about, inviting flies, and sometimes even dogs. Social activities, and even walking down a street had become terribly embarrassing. And then there were the fainting attacks. She was continuously dizzy. Her heart was always pounding, and so on, and so forth.

Deep down in her heart, Affiong concluded that her sister had cancer of the cervix. That was Affiong's specialty. The story was so typical of the ones she heard daily. Barring the familiar face, Eno was just like the patients she nursed every day. No wonder Kuffre had told her to start coming to Affiong. But attending to other people is one thing, attending to one's baby sister was another thing altogether. Affiong had begun to mourn her only sister already. Why was life so unfair? Eno had not even begun to live! Why, she had not even had the pleasures of a married person yet! Or had she? After all, cancer of the cervix is virtually unknown among nuns and life-time virgins.

She put the delicate question to Eno. Eno vehemently denied any form of sexual promiscuity.

At the house she only allowed Eno enough time to bath and freshen up. She took her to the hospital where she worked. Affiong called in many of her public relation debts. She cut through most of the red tapes. She made the doctors see her sister outside of their schedules, without prior appointments. If it were possible, she would have had her admitted into the cancer ward that same day and therapy commenced. The doctors put down their feet. They drew the line there. Her sister, they insisted, must have a Gynaecological review first. She must obtain a histological report, before being admitted as a cancer patient. Affiong saw the sense in this. Although she could also call in some debts in that department, the particular doctor that she wanted to see her sister had just finished clinic for that day. He would not run another one for the next five days. He counselled Affiong to be patient over the phone. "If your sister is really as bad as you say, a good dose of home care will probably do her more good than an impersonal hospital environment. Give her that comfort for a few more days. She might not enjoy that benefit again for a long time once she starts her treatments."

Affiong appreciated the sense in this and let up pressure. The delay would also give her enough opportunity to get re-acquainted with Eno. She would interview her more and sift out the facts for the doctors.

But what a long five days it was! Affiong experienced first-hand how it was to live with patients from whom such odours emanated. She would have eased her out of the house if not for the very close relationship with Eno. Besides, where else would she go? As it was, her husband and her children disdained coming home. They would stay away for as long as possible. One could easily tell that Eno had passed through a room. The smell would linger, after she had left for hours. Finally, she had to be moved into the boys' quarters and confined there. That way, at least the rest of the family could swallow their food.

When the five days were up, Affiong took Eno back to the hospital. She was determined that she should stay there till she had at least received some treatment. The doctor was very sympathetic. He took a lot of time clerking and examining Eno. When it was all over, he came out with what Affiong thought was an inappropriately big smile. "Congratulations!" he told Affiong, "It's not cancer after all!"

"What?" Affiong asked, quite dazed. "What do you mean it's not cancer after all? All the symptoms and signs are there!"

"Oh yes! But it is not cancer. What she has is a cervical polyp that has been bleeding, and is badly infected."

With recovering hope Affiong still begged, "Please don't tease me doctor. Be truthful with me."

"It's true" the doctor persisted. "I'm not teasing you."

"Then, what about the terrible odours? How come she is so emaciated?"

"It's the bleeding. Blood does have a terrible odour under certain circumstances. Don't get me wrong. This poor girl has been going through terrible times. She has lost so much blood. In fact, it's quite a wonder that she can still stand on her feet considering the amount of battle her systems are doing to combat anaemia and infections. She is even in heart failure. Her kidneys may be compromised as well. I suggest we admit her immediately, stabilize her, and then work her up for surgery. I expect a total recovery. We will, of course need many units of blood."

Blood? Only blood! Recounting the story so many years afterwards, Affiong never tired of telling how great a relief she felt. Had the doctor so much as asked for her parents' graves then, she would have gone to any length to get them. As it was, a few units of blood only required pressing a few buttons. She got her sons, her husband, and her brothers to come forward to be tested. They were all very willing to donate blood for Eno.

Eno did recover fully, not just physically, but also emotionally. She returned to her normal jolly self after that crisis. She had a new lease on life. About eighteen months after her ordeal, she married a very wonderful man that she had met on that fateful trip.

"I was just going to see my sister and then die!"

Today she is the mother of three lovely children. The children call Affiong "Mama", and call their own mom, "Aunty"!

Not That Inevitable

The reasons that people give for not wanting to go for cancer screening vary. The two commonest are that they are afraid that cancer might be found. They think it is for people that are too worried about their health. "If it is pregnancy," this second category says, "it will become very obvious one day." This is a foolish thing to say because by the time it becomes very obvious, it might also become too late to be treated.

Even health workers who know the benefit of these screening methods are also very reluctant to be screened. A look at this present story shows that just as "All that glitters is not gold", in the same vein, "All that is long is not a snake!" In fact, the long thing could even be a harmless rope or a useful cord.

Another reason people give is the inhibitory cost of screening. This is often very heavily subsidized, or even free through some philanthropies. Medical facilities can be quite expensive in some countries but what prize can one put on health? An Arab proverb says that health is "figure 1"; wealth, children, friends, position power, and every other thing human beings are ambitious for are just a string of zeros. Without health, all these things are just nothing. With good health however, they represent the joy of a lifetime!

When one has inexplicable symptoms, it is best to go to the hospital as soon as possible. At the best, a reassurance of good health could be obtained. At the worst, a dangerous disease will be caught on time before it gets out of hand.

That is POSITIVE ACTION!

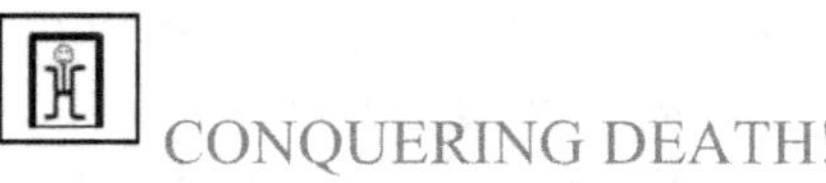CONQUERING DEATH!

– Isobel

If ever anybody lived a very eventful life, Isobel Kuhn did! Born Isobel Miller in 1901, and married to John Kuhn in 1928, she is now best remembered by the many inspiring and challenging books she wrote before she died. Two of the books – *By Searching*, and *In the Arena* were special autobiographies. She was born to a sickly mother that eventually died of cancer. She had a jolly father that was perpetually in debt.

Nevertheless, she grew up a socialite and loved to dance. When she was nineteen years she was spurned in love. She contemplated, but did not eventually attempt, suicide.

In the university, one of her professors challenged her belief in God. Isobel took a real introspective look at herself. She abandoned the faith she was taught as a child. She withdrew for a while from God. When eventually she made her tortuous way back to God "By Searching", she became very dedicated to Him. She decided to become a missionary. Against all odds, she traversed the continent, and went to school at Moody Bible Institute in Chicago.

After her studies, she went back to her native Vancouver. While keeping house for her father and her brother, she worked among the down-trodden and the hopeless. She brought them the message of hope. From there she eventually went to China to re-unite with John. They got married and were posted to work with the remote tribal Lisu people. Isobel was not much use as an itinerant travelling evangelist. She rather loved her role of staying to teach the Lisu, and to ground them in the faith. To them, she was their beloved Ma-ma.

During the Second World War, she became separated from her husband. John was the more "itinerant evangelist type". She was also separated from her little daughter who was away attending boarding school in a Japanese-held territory. She developed an abscessed tooth and was in severe pains. She was forced to travel away from the relative safety of the mountains to the Yunan area in China. She went by foot, by pack-animals, by rickety lorries, always one step ahead of danger.

Back to the mountains after the war, the communist threat began. Isobel and her young family were in constant danger of bandits, of diseases, of hostile soldiers, even of traitors among the people they had given their lives to serve. They learnt how to walk closer to God, and they experienced many of His miracles first-hand.

In 1950, under the new communist regime, all foreigners were forced to leave China. They had to abandon the people they had given sixteen years of their lives to and "escape" back to their native countries. This time, Isobel had to make the gruelling journey with her six-year-old son to boot. It might have been the height of sorrow and despondence, but they did not dwell long on it. There were still other places, other people groups that were still free and accessible. As an added bonus, there were native and displaced Lisu people living in Thailand. And so in 1952, the Khuns went to Thailand to continue their pioneering work. The children were left behind in

United States to complete their schooling. Isobel sorely missed them.

The Thai work was a pioneer work indeed. Although there had been missionary presence there for almost a century, it was centred mostly round the big cities. To reach the tribal peoples of the interior, the missionaries literally had to make the pathway to them. It was during one of these forays to the interior that Isobel got wounded in her breast. In her own words:

> *"We were walking single file, and a fallen tree branch lay concealed under the leaves of the path. As the young walker in front of me unknowingly stepped on one end, the other end sprang up and struck me severely..."[1]*

Back to civilization, the doctors said that it was only a torn ligament, but God ministered to Isobel that it was going to develop into a cancer. That injury would eventually cause her to return to America and her children. However, with the doctors' verdict, Isobel put it all out of her mind.

Seven months later, on another pioneering trip, Isobel slipped on mud. As she fell, a jagged tree stump hit her in the very same place she had been previously hit! X-rays were done and the doctors again reassured her. However, about two years after the initial incident, she noticed a lump in that breast. Initial biopsies said "Non-malignant". However, a more detailed study showed that it was malignant. Isobel had to undergo surgery first in Thailand, then in New York by 1954.

After her first surgery, Isobel was still in her hospital bed recovering. A senior doctor came to see her during a teaching ward round. He pointed out to his protégés how calm and serene she was. This was in contrast to some other patients. "It must have to do with being able to fix her mind on a force outside of herself" he said.

To this Isobel countered:

"Good psychology, certainly – he is quite a clever doctor. But how perfectly impossible for a person in such a weak condition to hook his faith on to some nebulae outside himself just

104

*because it would be to his benefit if he
could! That was not what I was doing! I was
resting back on a private word, spoken to me
two years before...*"[2]

She had a relationship with God even before
that sickness. The relationship merely continued.
That was what made the difference! She had her hard
days. She had times when she imagined terrible
things. However, she had a faith in God that ran
deeper than all that.

When it became obvious that the cancer was
not curable, Isobel retired to a quiet home in Illinois.
It had been given to the family by some friends.
Since she could not go back to her life's work, she
turned her hand to writing down her life experiences.
She disciplined herself to put in a certain quantity of
work each day. Out of this came the eight books that
have inspired so many up to now. As she told
friends, "These cancer years have been among my
happiest!"[3] She was not just trying to be brave or to
put on a face either.

She kept on writing till one day in 1957.
With trembling hands,

she pushed aside the papers and said, "I cannot write anymore!"[4] She turned to reading instead. About a month later she died. She was happy, fulfilled, and still inspiring people even after so many decades later!

1. In the Arena by Isobel Kuhn. China Inland Mission 1959. P. 182
2. Ibid. P. 185 - 186
3. One Vision Only by Carolyn Canfield. China Inland Mission. P. 187
4. Ibid. P187

Indomitable!

Oh Yes! Isobel Kuhn is one of my favourite authors. I have read all her eight books. I have also read a few others about her. I think that life is aimless unless one finds a cause to live for; set goals to achieve and do what one feels called to do. That is what Isobel's By Searching is mostly about. Those that search really find. What I admire most about her is the ability to make the most out of every situation. It could be a dysfunctional home, problems at school, waiting impatiently for an overseas posting, struggling with learning a foreign language and culture, being left alone in a hostile environment, struggling with cancer, or whatever! Isobel always found some way of facing whatever it was with the perspective of her calling in God. She even found some ways to inject some humour into every situation or circumstance.

While writing this book, I met Hajiya Fati. She has also been suffering from cancer of the breast. She has had two operations so far. Right now, she suffers from a very swollen and painful right arm and hand as a result of the second operation. She is never shy nor tired of sharing her experiences, and her struggles in coping with cancer as long as it would be of benefit to someone. She always ended by saying, "If I had died two years ago, the cancer would really have got me. However, knowing that I had this terrible disease gave me the impetus to work very hard to finish my doctorate program. At least if I die now, my obituary would read Dr. Fati..."

Now, is that not an indomitable spirit?

For those that read this but do not have cancer, what are you working for? What are you living for? Find your goal, find your focus in life. Go for it! Live now as if there might not be much time left. There might not be.

To my friend Cheryl Hill:

STILL, YOU ***ARE*** A BRIGHT FLAME!

– We still remember

APPENDIX

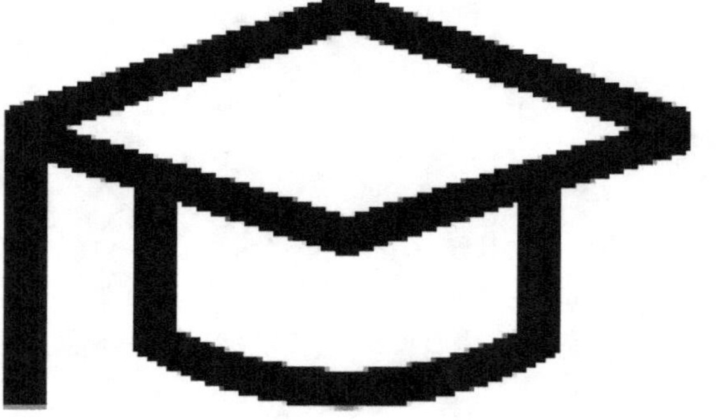

<u>WHAT IS CANCER?</u>

Cancer is a group of diseases in which a single cell or a group of cells begin to grow independent of the body control mechanisms, to the detriment of the other body organs, and the individual as a whole.

Every living tissue in the body is always growing, dying and being replaced, or being repaired after a damage. Every living tissue in the body is therefore capable of developing cancer. That means there can be cancer of the skin, of the nerves, of the bones, of the womb, of the intestines and so on.

Experts tell us that many cancerous (rebellious) tissues start developing in our bodies every day. However, the body defence mechanisms are usually able to take care of and put out most of them. Under some conditions, this control mechanism is lost, overwhelmed, not efficient enough, or becomes "deceived". That is how cancer develops.

All the mechanisms that lead to the development of cancer are still poorly understood. The miracle is that we do not develop cancer more often!

<u>WHAT CAUSES CANCER?</u>

A better question should actually be: why does the body mechanism fail, and cancer allowed to develop?

Again, this is not quite well understood. Broadly speaking however, the reasons can be divided into two groups: something that one is born with; and some sort of "insult" from the environment.

IN-BORN FACTORS

Some people are born with some cells that are abnormal right from the beginning. These cells just wait like a timed bomb to explode. For years, they may just lie dormant, or be growing in a manner that is not quickly noticeable. When they finally do "explode", it may be in infancy like some childhood cancers of the eye, the blood or the brain. It may be during adolescence like some blood cancers, and especially some cancers of the testes or the ovaries. It could also be much later in life.

These days, people are living much longer than before. Whereas other things might have killed them in the past before their cancers manifest, with improved medical care, they live long enough for the abnormal cancer cells to manifest.

It is also thought that some people are born, inadequately equipped to combat the day-to-day assaults against the body. These assaults include developing cancer cells. Sooner or later, their body defence mechanisms become overwhelmed, and cancer develops. This would explain why cancer tends to run in some families. A grandmother may have had cancer of the breast, the mother cancer of the ovaries, a sister cancer of the intestines, and a daughter cancer of the womb and so on.

ENVIRONMENTAL "INSULTS"

Repeated insults to the body tend to result in cancer. Again, it is not fully understood how this comes about. It could be that the body gets used to the repeated insults and just tolerates it to its own detriment. It could also be that the defence mechanisms get overwhelmed, and cancer can no longer be prevented. It might also be that the cells that were "woken up" to take care of the insults just refuse to go back to sleep again. In continuing to work they slip out of the control of the rest of the body and become cancer cells.

There are different kinds of insults, but a major grouping would include the following:

Infections: Viruses are specially the culprits here. The Hepatitis B Virus (HBV) is known to cause liver cancer. The Human Papilloma Virus (HPV) causes cancer of the cervix. The Human Immuno deficiency Virus (HIV) causes a type of skin cancer. The Epstein Barr Virus causes blood and lymph node cancers and so on.

Other organisms like the plasmodium that causes malaria is related to a type of blood and jaw cancer. The bladder fluke is related to cancer of the bladder. The liver fluke is related to liver cancer.

Chemical Poisons: The commonest poison that has been confirmed to cause cancer is the tobacco break-down products in cigarettes. Not only do they cause cancer of the lungs, they make it more likely for an individual to develop other kinds of cancers – like cancer of the cervix or the stomach, besides other diseases   that are not cancers!

The association is so strong that people that do not smoke themselves but are constantly in the company of those that do, also stand a higher risk of developing cancer. Again, stopping to smoke drastically reduces this risk. The risks begin to reverse once the person stops smoking, though never completely.

Other chemicals that are known to cause cancer include Coal dust and asbestos dust in those that work in the mines or factories. Petro-chemicals, some textile dyes, and lead are also culprits. Aflatoxin is a kind of chemical found in stored nuts (like groundnuts) that have been infected by blight (a type of fungus). Infections might be destroyed by the prolonged heat of boiling. Toxins only become more concentrated. If that food looks spoiled, throw it away!

Every medication has potential side effects. Some medications can cause cancer or enhance its formation in one way or another. Fortunately, most of them are labelled as "Very Dangerous Medications" and can usually only be obtained by a doctor's prescription. Doctors prescribe them only when the benefits are known to far out-weigh the potential risks.

Trauma: Physical trauma is known to provoke cancer formation, especially when it occurs repeatedly, and is to the same part of the body. Continuous exposure to sunlight is known to provoke cancer of the skin, especially in albinos. A man has been known to develop cancer of the breast because the belt of his braces was always chaffing the skin around his breast. Some women develop different sorts of cancer, from wearing tight corsets, belts, or brassieres with stays.

Repeated surgeries, especially cosmetic surgeries, have also been fingered as a cause of cancer. This is perhaps due to the fact that the healing cells are being unnecessarily over-stretched.

<u>HOW DOES CANCER MANIFEST?</u>

The manifestation of a cancer will depend on several factors. Do the cells that are multiplying out of control have a specific function in the body? Are the cancer cells blocking the function of any other important organ as they grow? Has the growth of the cancer reached the outside where it can be felt or seen? Have the cancer cells been carried to other areas of the body where the effect is more quickly noticed?

The person that has cancer begins to emaciate as the body stores are taken over by the growing cancer cells. In fact, the very first sign of cancer may be an increasing tiredness, weakness, and pallor. By the time the person loses a lot of weight, the cancer is probably at its terminal stages.

If the cancer cells have a specific function in the body, this function becomes exaggerated. Cancer of the womb, or cervix may come with increasing discharge. Cancer of the thyroids may come with excessive heat. Cancer of the adrenal glands may present with excessive thirst.

When vital organs like the urinary tracts are blocked, the person is unable to make or to pass urine. If the throat is blocked, the person finds it difficult to swallow and always feels as if there is something that is refusing to go down. If it blocks the airways, breathing and talking become difficult, and so on.

Most cancers will cause swelling that may be felt under the skin. Some even grow beyond the containing skin to form a sore. Any sore that refuses to heal quickly should be checked for cancer at once.

Some cancers, their deposits, or seedlings, can also "eat into" vital organs. When they eat into the bladder or the anus, the individual will continually leak urine or faeces. If they eat into a major blood vessel, internal bleeding will occur. This author has seen a cancer in the nose that ate into the mouth so that the young man could not talk clearly without first pinching close the nose to prevent air escaping as he talked.

Because it is the same blood that circulates to all parts of the body, cancer from one part can get carried to another part.

118

This is called "METASTASIS". Metastasis to the lungs, the brain, or the liver are considered the most terminal stages of the disease. In **most** cases this spells inevitable death. In some rare cases, a cure can still be achieved, even at this late stage.

Cancer can also present with the sign of where it has metastasized to. Severe headaches and even mental problems may manifest when it has reached the brain. Coughing out blood and difficulty in breathing will manifest when it has reached the lungs. When it has reached the liver there are a wide range of difficulties. Cancers of the different components of blood have so many different ways of manifesting that they will deserve another book by themselves.

<u>HOW DOES CANCER KILL?</u>

Cancer has several ways of finally causing the individual to die. In the first instance, just by taking over the body's stores and depriving all other organs and tissues of essential nutrients, it keeps weakening the individual till the person is virtually starved to death.

Cancer also directs all the body mechanism towards fighting it. This means that other challenges that the individual faces on a daily basis go unaddressed. Infections, fevers, even a minor trauma might be what finally leads to the death of the person.

As they grow rapidly, so they also die rapidly. If the body clean-up systems are not able to cope, the cancer waste products accumulate in the body. They become poisonous to the systems, causing death.

Cancer cells also have a habit of breaking off and entering the blood streams as small solid masses. Mostly these can quickly be turned into liquid that the body can carry. If not, as it reaches the brain, it can cause paralysis. It if it reaches organs like the heart or the lungs, it can cause instant death.

Cancers can also block some vital organs in its function, choking off blood supply. It might also cause internal bleeding. If these are not met head-on as grave emergencies the individual will surely die. Incidentally, such things happen when the individual is not even fit for surgery. Taken in for surgery for such an emergency, it may be the stress of the surgery that will finally do the deed.

Every form of treatment has its own risks and hazards. Some patients may die in the course of treatment. Any treatment option is usually weighed. The doctors, the patients, and their relatives must be satisfied that the potential benefits far out-weigh the potential risks before embarking on any treatment or treatment combinations.

<u>CAN CANCER BE TREATED?</u>

Treatment aims for cancers can be divided into two: Curative and Palliative. Adjuvant treatments apply to both.

Curative treatments are aimed at totally taking away the disease. Palliative treatment means that even though the disease cannot be totally cured at the stage it has reached, something can still be done to reduce its effects to make it more bearable. It would improve the individual's quality of life.

Adjuvant treatments are all the other things that are done for the patient to enable him or her fight the disease. It would also help the person live out the remaining days in ease and comfort in palliative treatments. Adjuvant treatments equip the body to continue fighting. Most adjuvant treatments would include reasonable diets, blood building or supplementations, and pain killers.

Palliative and curative treatments are much along the same lines but the approach to palliative treatment is less harsh and less radical since the aim is not really to cure. Thus, operations done at this stage is more or less just to remove dead or smelly tissues, not the cancer itself. Radiotherapy may be just to stop bleeding, not to kill off the cancer cells, and so on.

DEVELOPING METHODS

Some experimental methods for treating cancer are still under research. As at now, the following are the common methods:

Surgery: Operations done to either remove the cancer or the region of the body where the cancer is found like the breast, a limb, or the intestines. Sometimes, the aim is not to remove the cancer totally, but to remove the bulk of it, and shrink it to a size that can be managed by other forms of treatment.

Chemotherapy: This has to do with the administration of medications. These could be in the form of tablets, capsules, injections, and infusions. These medications are very powerful medications. They are supposed to be poisonous. Unfortunately they affect not just to the cancer cells, but also other actively growing cells of the body such as the blood, skin, and hair tissues. Their side-effects are therefore felt along such lines.

Hormonal Treatments: Some of the medications that are used are also hormones, their analogues or their antagonists. This is especially so in cancers of the breasts, the womb, the prostate etc. Hormonal treatments also involve the removal of, or the incapacitation of the major organs from which the hormones that supports the cancer growth is produced. The ovaries, the testes, the adrenals, the thyroid, the pancreas and so on could be removed.

Radiotherapy: This involves the treatment of cancer with ionizing radiations. These are the same substances that are used to make the atomic bomb. They are not to be handled carelessly. It is an example of an event of the good that can come out of evil. Every country has only a few well-guarded centres where this kind of treatments can be done.

Immuno-therapy, stem cell therapy, hyperthermia etc.: These are methods that are not yet widely in use. Some are still being researched and undergoing trials. The results so far are very encouraging.

Diet: Since writing this, I had been approached about the use of diet to treat cancer. The diet that has been talked about is a wholly vegetarian diet of mostly natural fruit and vegetable juices. It involves a shunning of all animal products including milk and eggs. It is also often accompanied with life-style changes such as increased exercise and fresh air.

I have no doubt that there are unorthodox methods that would work in cancer treatment, and other disease treatment for that matter. I have humbly acknowledged that medical science does not have all the answers. Researches are still ongoing in many areas. The things that have been written here are those that we know for now, in this field. Be careful though, of what you choose to adopt. At the end of your rope, a desperate choice could save you. My counsel is: "Be wise!"

<u>CAN CANCER BE PREVENTED?</u>

Cancer can definitely be prevented if one knew the direction it was coming from.

Primary level prevention includes lifestyle changes that would prevent external insults. For instance, albinos should use sunscreen, wear broad hats, and use umbrellas when out in the sunlight. people that work with dangerous chemicals should wear protective clothing. Mosquito bites should be avoided by all means. Wherever possible, immunizations against viral infections should be taken. Other such measures would definitely help.

Smoking and smokers should be avoided. Foods that have been contaminated should be discarded or destroyed. Incidentally, chemical toxins only get more concentrated, and therefore more deadly when heated.

When all known factors have been avoided, the rest is to take one's chances with living a normal life. Experts advise on balanced diets and exercise as a mode of preventing cancer. Both of these help the immune system (our in-born defence systems) to keep working maximally. The same experts also advise against over-eating and obesity. These have also been implicated in cancer development.

Good advice is: DO ALL THINGS IN MODERATION.

For secondary level prevention, people should take advantage of cancer screening programs including PAP smears, mammograms, colonoscopies, prostate screen, and so on. Some examinations can even be done at home like Breast Self-Examination (BSE). See the following portion.

It is very important that every ill-health that lasts longer that two days be checked out by a doctor. When one doctor becomes stumped, another doctor's opinion should be sought, complete with the appropriate letters of reference. This second doctor should of course preferably be a specialist in the field concerned.

Any hint of a cancer should be fully and adequately treated as soon as the diagnosis is made, with the aim of achieving a cure. The worst that could happen is to be laughed at, and called names like "Hypochondriac", or "Paranoid". It is better to be called those names than to die in silence of a deadly disease!

Tertiary level prevention would involve getting back to as near normal a life as possible, and making the most of whatever is left of it. For some people, it may involve the procurement of prosthesis – artificial limbs and such. The prostheses made these days look so natural that unless one is told, it might not even be easy to distinguish from the natural body part.

CANCER SCREENING PROGRAMS

Screening programs are meant for those who do not have any sign of the disease at all, but are at increased risk of developing it. There are several packages that are available now. Some are even subsidized by various non-governmental organizations. All are supported by governments in one way or another. PAP smear and culposcopy for cervical cancer screening are available, as well as mammography for breast cancer screening.

Every woman should know how to do breast self-examination at a given time every month. She should know the abnormalities to look for. If any abnormality is detected, she should also know how, and to whom, it should be reported.

It is well worth the while to have a general medical examination from time to time in one's lifetime. Cancer screening should be a part of this.

In these series, Dr. I. C. Ozed-Williams draws from a vast experience of working with women as an Obstetrician-Gynaecologist, a Community Counsellor, and as a woman herself.

Dr. Ozed-Williams is a Fellow of both the West African College of Surgeons and The International College of surgeons but writes with a lot of simplicity that will both intrigue and benefit a layman as well as the seasoned professional. These books are well worth reading.

OTHER BOOKS IN THIS SERIES

THE TALES OF TEN WOMEN (*Fibroids)*
THE BATTLES OF TEN WOMEN (*Cancer*)
THE BURDENS OF TEN WOMEN (*Infertility*)
THE SORROWS OF TEN WOMEN (*Losing Unborn Babies)*
TEN WOMEN IN TROUBLE (*Dying in Childbirth*)
TEN WOMEN IN JOYOUS PAIN (*Operative Deliveries*)